Healthy Keto Vegetarian Lifestyle

Tasty Easy Recipes to Increase your Energy and Lose Weight

Ricardo Abagnale

Table of Contents

INTRODUCTION 6

BREAKFAST 7

    ALMOND FLOUR WAFFLES.. 7

    HEALTHY BREAKFAST PORRIDGE... 9

MAINS 11

    CREAMY ONION SOUP... 11

    BAKED ZUCCHINI EGGPLANT WITH CHEESE.................................. 13

    ZUCCHINI HUMMUS.. 15

    ARTICHOKE DIP... 17

    CRUSTLESS VEGGIE QUICHE 19

    AVOCADO CILANTRO DIP 21

    EGG SALAD 23

    EGG STUFFED CUCUMBER...25

    CARAMELIZED ENDIVE WITH GARLIC..27

SIDES..29

    MUSHROOMS AND BLACK BEANS 29

    BROCCOLI WITH BRUSSELS SPROUTS 31

    GLAZED CAULIFLOWER..33

    GARLIC ASPARAGUS AND TOMATOES..35

    HOT CUCUMBER MIX...37

    TOMATO SALAD 39

FRUIT AND VEGETABLES 41

    MINTED PEAS FETA RICE... 41

    HEARTY BABY CARROTS..43

    SENSITIVE STEAMED ARTICHOKES 45

    RHUBARB AND STRAWBERRY COMPOTE 47

Zucchini Cakes 49

SOUPS AND STEWS 51

Two-Potato Soup with Rainbow Chard 51

Hot & Sour Tofu Soup 53

Autumn Medley Stew 56

KETO PASTA 59

Garlic-Butter Tempeh with Shirataki Fettucine 59

Eggplant Ragu 62

SALADS 65

Corn and Red Bean Salad 65

Greek Potato Salad 67

Rainbow Quinoa Salad.. 69

SNACKS 71

Veggie Spread... 71

Pomegranate Dip 73

Tomato and Watermelon Bites 75

Artichoke and Spinach Salad 77

Red Pepper and Cheese Dip.. 79

Mushroom Falafel... 81

DESSERTS 83

Mango Rice Pudding 83

Tapioca with Apricots.. 85

Poached Pears in Ginger Sauce 87

Baked Apples 89

Maple & Rum Apples 91

Pumpkin & Chocolate Loaf 93

Cheesecake 95

GLUTEN-FREE NUTELLA BROWNIE TRIFLE..97

OTHER RECIPES **99**

CHINESE SOUP AND GINGER SAUCE...99

CORN CREAM SOUP 102

VEGGIE MEDLEY...104

LENTILS CURRY 106

LENTILS DAL 108

FRUIT DISH 110

INTRODUCTION

The Ketogenic diet is truly life changing. The diet improves your overall health and helps you lose the extra weight in a matter of days. The diet will show its multiple benefits even from the beginning and it will become your new lifestyle really soon.

As soon as you embrace the Ketogenic diet, you will start to live a completely new life.

On the other hand, the vegetarian diet is such a healthy dietary option you can choose when trying to live healthy and also lose some weight.

The collection we bring to you today is actually a combination between the Ketogenic and vegetarian diets. You get to discover some amazing Ketogenic vegetarian dishes you can prepare in the comfort of your own home. All the dishes you found here follow both the Ketogenic and the vegetarian rules, they all taste delicious and rich and they are all easy to make.

We can assure you that such a combo is hard to find. So, start a keto diet with a vegetarian "touch" today. It will be both useful and fun!

So, what are you still waiting for? Get started with the Ketogenic diet and learn how to prepare the best and most flavored Ketogenic vegetarian dishes. Enjoy them all!

Almond Flour Waffles

Preparation time: 10 minutes

Cooking time: 5 minutes

Servings: 2

Nutritional Values (Per Serving):

- Calories: 208
- Fat: 18 g
- Carbohydrates: 4.83 g
- Sugar: 2.1 g
- Protein: 6.52 g
- Cholesterol: 114 mg

Ingredients:

- Pinch of xanthan gum
- Pinch of salt
- 1 tablespoon butter, melted
- 1 large organic egg
- 2 tablespoons sour cream
- 1 teaspoon vinegar

- 2 teaspoons arrowroot flour
- 1/8 teaspoon baking powder 1/8 teaspoon baking soda
- ¼ cup almond flour

Directions:

1. In a mixing bowl combine vinegar, butter, sour cream, and egg mix well.
2. Add dry ingredients into wet and mix until well blended.
3. Heat your waffle iron and cook waffle for 5 minutes or to your waffle iron instructions.
4. Serve and enjoy!

Healthy Breakfast Porridge

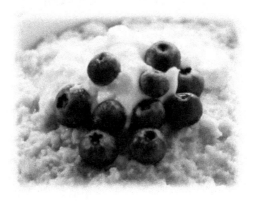

Preparation time: 5 minutes

Cooking time: 5 minutes

Servings: 2

Nutritional Values (Per Serving):

- Calories: 222
- Fat: 21 g
- Carbohydrates: 3.90 g
- Sugar: 3.9 g
- Protein: 2.68 g,
- Cholesterol: 49 mg

Ingredients:

- 1/8 teaspoon salt

- 4 tablespoons coconut, unsweetened, shredded
- 1 tablespoon oat bran
- 1 tablespoon flaxseed meal
- ½ tablespoon butter
- ¾ teaspoon Truvia
- ½ teaspoon cinnamon
- ½ cup heavy cream
- 1 cup water

Directions:

1. Add all your ingredients into a saucepan over medium-low heat. Once the mixture comes to a boil remove from heat.
2. Serve warm and enjoy!

Creamy Onion Soup

Preparation time: 15 minutes

Cooking time: 25 minutes

Servings: 4

Nutritional Values (Per Serving):

- Calories: 90
- Sugar: 4.1 g
- Fat: 7.4 g
- Carbohydrates: 10.1 g
- Cholesterol: 0 mg
- Protein: 1 g

Ingredients:

- 1 shallot, sliced Sea salt
- 1 ½ tablespoons extra-virgin olive oil

- 1 leek, sliced
- 1 garlic clove, chopped
- 4 cups vegetable stock
- 1 onion, sliced

Directions:

1. Add the olive oil and vegetable stock into a large saucepan over medium heat, bring to a boil.
2. Add the remaining ingredients and stir. Cover and simmer for 25 minutes.
3. Puree your soup using a blender until smooth.
4. Serve warm and enjoy!

Baked Zucchini Eggplant with Cheese

Preparation time: 15 minutes

Cooking time: 35 minutes

Servings: 6

Nutritional Values (Per Serving):

- Calories: 110
- Cholesterol: 10 mg
- Carbohydrates: 10.4 g
- Fat: 5.8 g
- Sugar:4.8 g
- Protein: 7 g

Ingredients:

- 3-ounces Parmesan cheese, grated
- 3 medium zucchinis, sliced

- 1 tablespoon extra-virgin olive oil
- 1 medium eggplant, sliced
- 1 cup cherry tomatoes, halved
- ¼ cup parsley, chopped
- ¼ cup basil, chopped
- 4 garlic cloves, minced
- ¼ teaspoon sea salt
- ¼ teaspoon pepper

Directions:

1. Preheat your oven to 350°Fahrenheit. Spray a baking dish with cooking spray.
2. In a mixing bowl, add eggplant, cherry tomatoes, zucchini, olive oil, cheese, basil, garlic, salt, and pepper, toss to mix.
3. Transfer eggplant mixture to baking dish and place into preheated oven to bake for 35 minutes.
4. Garnish with chopped parsley. Serve and enjoy!

Zucchini Hummus

Preparation time: 10 minutes

Cooking time: 10 minutes

Servings: 4

Nutritional Values (Per Serving):

- Calories: 138
- Cholesterol: 0 mg
- Sugar: 4.9 g
- Fat: 10.1 g
- Carbohydrates: 11.1 g
- Protein: 4.6 g

Ingredients:

- 3 garlic cloves
- 4 zucchinis, halved
- 3 tablespoons tahini

- 1 tablespoon extra-virgin olive oil
- 1 tablespoon lemon juice, fresh
- 1 teaspoon cumin
- ¼ cup cilantro, chopped
- Pepper and salt to taste

Directions:

1. Place your zucchini onto the grill. Season zucchini with salt and pepper. Grill for 10 minutes.
2. Add grilled zucchini, lemon juice, cilantro, cumin, tahini, garlic, olive oil, salt, and pepper into a blender and blend until smooth.
3. Pour the zucchini mixture into serving bowl.
4. Sprinkle top with paprika. Serve and enjoy!

Artichoke Dip

Preparation time: 5 minutes

Cooking time: 35 minutes

Servings: 4

Nutritional Values (Per Serving):

- Calories: 284
- Fat: 19.4 g
- Cholesterol: 37 mg
- Sugar: 3.8 g
- Carbohydrates: 19 g
- Protein: 11.2 g

Ingredients:

- 15-ounces artichoke hearts, drained
- 1 cup cheddar cheese, shredded
- 3 cups arugula, chopped
- 1 teaspoon Worcestershire sauce

- ½ cup mayonnaise
- 1 tablespoon onion, minced

Directions:

1. Preheat your oven to 350° Fahrenheit.
2. Blend all ingredients using a blender and blend until smooth.
3. Pour artichoke mixture into a baking dish and bake in preheated oven for 30 minutes.
4. Serve with crackers and enjoy!

Crustless Veggie Quiche

Preparation time: 10 minutes

Cooking time: 30 minutes

Servings: 6

Nutritional Values (Per Serving):

- Calories: 257
- Sugar: 4.2 g
- Fat: 16.7 g
- Carbohydrates: 8.1 g
- Cholesterol: 257 mg
- Protein: 21.4 g

Ingredients:

- 1 cup milk
- 1 cup tomatoes, chopped
- 1 cup Parmesan cheese, grated, fresh
- 1 onion, chopped

- 1 cup zucchini, chopped
- 8 eggs, organic
- ½ teaspoon pepper
- 1 teaspoon sea salt

Directions:

1. Preheat your oven to 400°Fahrenheit.
2. In a pan placed over medium heat, melt butter, add onion and sauté until lightly brown. Add zucchini and tomatoes to pan and sauté for 5 minutes.
3. Beat eggs with milk, cheese, pepper and salt in a bowl. Pour egg mixture over veggies and bake in preheated oven for 30 minutes.
4. Allow dish to cool for 10 minutes, cut into slices, serve and enjoy!

Avocado Cilantro Dip

Preparation time: 10 minutes

Servings: 2

Nutritional Values (Per Serving):

- Calories: 273
- Cholesterol: 13 mg
- Sugar: 2.1 g
- Fat: 25.7 g
- Carbohydrates: 11.6 g
- Protein: 3 g

Ingredients:

- 1 cup cilantro, fresh
- 1 garlic clove
- ½ cup sour cream
- ½ teaspoon onion powder
- 1 fresh lemon juice

- 2 avocados
- ¼ teaspoon sea salt

Directions:

1. Using your blender blend ingredients, and blend until smooth.
2. Place the mixture in your fridge to combine flavors for a few hours.
3. Serve with crackers and enjoy!

Egg Salad

Preparation time: 15 minutes

Servings: 4

Nutritional Values (Per Serving):

- Calories: 80
- Sugar: 1.7 g
- Fat: 4.7 g
- Carbohydrates: 2.6 g
- Cholesterol: 165 mg
- Protein: 6.8 g

Ingredients:

- 4 eggs, organic, hard-boiled
- 1 teaspoon Dijon mustard
- ¾ cup celery, diced
- ¼ teaspoon pepper
- 1 tablespoon dill, fresh, chopped

- ¼ cup plain yogurt
- ½ teaspoon salt

Directions:

1. Peel your hard-boiled eggs and dice in a large mixing bowl.
2. Add celery, yogurt, dill, pepper, and salt. Mix well.
3. Serve and enjoy!

Egg Stuffed Cucumber

Preparation time: 15 minutes

Servings: 4

Nutritional Values (Per Serving):

Calories: 89

Sugar: 2.8 g

Fat: 4.8 g

Carbohydrates: 4.6 g

Cholesterol: 165 mg

Protein: 7.1 g

Ingredients:

- 1 large cucumber
- 2 tablespoons parsley, chopped
- 2 teaspoons Dijon mustard

- 1/8 teaspoon cayenne pepper
- ¼ cup plain yogurt
- 1 celery stalk, diced
- 4 eggs, organic, hard-boiled, peeled
- 1/8 teaspoon sea salt

Directions:

1. In a bowl mash your eggs using a fork.
2. Add into bowl celery, parsley, mustard, yogurt, pepper and salt and stir well.
3. Slice cucumber in half then cut each piece in half lengthwise. Scoop out cucumber seeds. Stuff with egg mixture the four cucumber boats.
4. Sprinkle tops with cayenne pepper. Serve and enjoy!

Caramelized Endive with Garlic

Preparation time: 10 minutes

Cooking time: 22 minutes

Servings: 8

Nutritional Values (Per Serving):

- Calories: 105
- Cholesterol: 0 mg
- Sugar: 0.6 g
- Fat: 7.3 g
- Carbohydrates: 9.2 g
- Protein: 3.3 g

- **Ingredients:**
- 2 tablespoons shallots, sliced
- 4 heads endive, sliced in half
- 1 teaspoon garlic, chopped
- ¼ teaspoon pepper

- ¼ cup coconut oil
- ½ teaspoon sea salt

Directions:

1. Melt the coconut oil in a pan over low heat. Once it has melted add shallots, and garlic and cook for 2 minutes. Place endive in the pan and cook for 20 minutes on low heat.
2. Season with salt and pepper. Serve and enjoy!

Mushrooms and Black Beans

Preparation time: 10 minutes

Cooking time: 25 minutes

Servings: 4

Nutritional Values (Per Serving):

- Calories 189
- Fat 3
- Fiber 4
- Carbs 9
- Protein 8

Ingredients:

- 1 pound mushrooms, sliced
- 1 yellow onion, chopped
- 1 teaspoon cumin, ground

- 1 teaspoon sweet paprika
- 1 cup canned black beans, drained and rinsed
- 2 tablespoons olive oil
- ½ cup chicken stock
- A pinch of salt and black pepper
- 2 tablespoons cilantro, chopped

Directions:

1. Heat up a pan with the oil over medium heat, add the onion and sauté for 5 minutes.
2. Add the mushrooms and sauté for 5 minutes more.
3. Add the rest of the ingredients, toss, cook over medium heat for 15 minutes more.
4. Divide everything between plates and serve as a side dish.

Broccoli with Brussels Sprouts

Preparation time: 10 minutes

Cooking time: 25 minutes

Servings: 4

Nutritional Values (Per Serving):

- calories 129
- fat 7.6
- fiber 5.3
- carbs 13.7
- protein 5.2

Ingredients:

- 1 pound broccoli florets
- ½ pound Brussels sprouts, trimmed and halved
- 2 tablespoons olive oil
- 1 tablespoon ginger, grated

- 1 tablespoon balsamic vinegar
- A pinch of salt and black pepper

Directions:

1. In a roasting pan, combine the broccoli with the sprouts and the other ingredients, toss gently and bake at 380 degrees F for 25 minutes.
2. Divide the mix between plates and serve.

Glazed Cauliflower

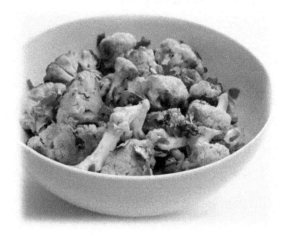

Preparation time: 10 minutes

Cooking time: 25 minutes

Servings: 4

Nutritional Values (Per Serving):

- Calories 76
- Fat 3.9
- Fiber 3.4
- Carbs 10.3
- Protein 2.4

Ingredients:

- 1 tablespoon olive oil
- 1 pound cauliflower florets
- 1 tablespoon maple syrup
- 1 tablespoon rosemary, chopped
- A pinch of salt and black pepper
- 1 teaspoon chili powder

Directions:

1. Spread the cauliflower on a baking sheet lined with parchment paper, add the oil and the other ingredients, toss and cook in the oven at 375 degrees F for 25 minutes.
2. Divide the mix between plates and serve.

Garlic Asparagus and Tomatoes

Preparation time: 10 minutes

Cooking time: 20 minutes

Servings: 4

Nutritional Values (Per Serving):

- Calories 132
- Fat 1
- Fiber 2
- Carbs 4
- Protein 4

Ingredients:

- 1 pound asparagus, trimmed and halved
- ½ pound cherry tomatoes, halved
- 2 tablespoons olive oil
- 1 teaspoon turmeric powder
- 2 tablespoons shallot, chopped

- A pinch of salt and black pepper
- 1 tablespoon chives, chopped

Directions:

1. Spread the asparagus on a baking sheet lined with parchment paper, add the tomatoes and the other ingredients, toss, cook in the oven at 375 degrees F for 20 minutes.
2. Divide everything between plates and serve as a side dish.

Hot Cucumber Mix

Preparation time: 10 minutes

Cooking time: 0 minutes

Servings: 4

Nutritional Values (Per Serving):

- Calories 132
- Fat 3
- Fiber 1
- Carbs 7
- Protein 4

Ingredients:

- 1 pound cucumbers, sliced
- 1 tablespoon olive oil
- 1 teaspoon chili powder
- 1 green chili, chopped
- 1 garlic clove, minced

- 1 tablespoon dill, chopped
- 2 tablespoons lime juice
- 1 tablespoon balsamic vinegar

Directions:

1. In a bowl, combine the cucumbers with the garlic, the oil and the other ingredients, toss and serve as a side salad.

Tomato Salad

Preparation time: 10 minutes

Cooking time: 0 minutes

Servings: 4

Nutritional Values (Per Serving):

- Calories 180
- Fat 2
- Fiber 2
- Carbs 8
- Protein 6

Ingredients:

- 1 pound cherry tomatoes, halved
- 3 scallions, chopped
- 1 tablespoon olive oil
- A pinch of salt and black pepper

- 1 tablespoon lime juice
- ¼ cup parsley, chopped

Directions:

2. In a bowl, combine the tomatoes with the scallions and the other ingredients, toss and serve as a side salad.

Minted Peas Feta Rice

Preparation time: 15 mins

Servings: 2

Nutritional Values (Per Serving):

- Calories: 28.1
- Fat:18.2 g
- Carbs:10.3 g
- Protein:8.8 g
- Sugars:2.2 g
- Sodium:216 mg

Ingredients:

- 1 ¼ c. vegetable broth
- ¾ c. brown rice
- ¼ c. finely crumbled feta cheese

- ¾ c. sliced scallions
- 1 ½ c. frozen peas
- Freshly ground pepper
- ¼ c. sliced fresh mint

Directions:

1. Boil broth in a saucepan over medium heat.
2. Add rice and bring it to a simmer. Cook for 4 minutes.
3. Stir in peas and cook for 6 minutes.
4. Turn off the heat then add feta, mint, scallions, and pepper.
5. Serve warm.

Hearty Baby Carrots

Preparation time: 5 mins

Servings: 4

Nutritional Values (Per Serving):

- Calories: 131
- Fat:10 g
- Carbs:11 g
- Protein:1 g
- Sugars:5 g
- Sodium:190 mg

Ingredients:

- 1 tbsp. chopped fresh mint
- 1 c. water
- Sea flavored vinegar
- 1 lb. baby carrots
- 1 tbsp. clarified ghee

Directions:

1. Place a steamer rack on top of your pot and add the carrots
2. Add water
3. Lock up the lid and cook at HIGH pressure for 2 minutes
4. Do a quick release
5. Pass the carrots through a strainer and drain them
6. Wipe the insert clean
7. Return the insert to the pot and set the pot to Sauté mode
8. Add clarified butter and allow it to melt
9. Add mint and sauté for 30 seconds
10. Add carrots to the insert and sauté well
11. Remove them and sprinkle with bit of flavored vinegar on top
12. Enjoy!

Sensitive Steamed Artichokes

Preparation time: 5 mins

Servings: 4

Nutritional Values (Per Serving):

- Calories: 77
- Fat:5 g
- Carbs:0 g
- Protein:2 g
- Sugars:1.3 g
- Sodium:121 mg

Ingredients:

- 1 halved lemon
- ¼ tsp. paprika
- 2 tbsps. Homemade Whole30 mayo
- 2 medium artichokes
- 1 tsp. Dijon mustard

Directions:

1. Wash the artichokes and remove the damaged outer leaves
2. Trim the spines and cut off upper edge
3. Wipe the cur edges with lemon half
4. Slice the stem and peel the stem
5. Chop it up and keep them on the side
6. Add a cup of water to the pot and place a steamer basket inside
7. Transfer the artichokes to the steamer basket and a squeeze of lemon
8. Lock up the lid and cook on HIGH pressure for 10 minutes
9. Release the pressure naturally
10. Enjoy

Rhubarb and Strawberry Compote

Preparation time: 10 mins

Servings: 4

Nutritional Values (Per Serving):

- Calories: 41.1
- Fat:2.1 g
- Carbs:5.5 g
- Protein:1.4 g
- Sugars:12 g
- Sodium:2.4 mg

Ingredients:

- 3 tbsps. Date paste
- ½ c. water Fresh mint
- 2 lbs. rhubarb
- 1 lb. strawberries

Directions:

1. Peel the rhubarb using a paring knife and chop it up ½ inch pieces

2. Add the chopped up rhubarb to your pot alongside water

3. Lock up the lid and cook on HIGH pressure for 10 minutes

4. Stem and quarter your strawberries and keep them on the side

5. Add the strawberries and date paste, give it a nice stir

6. Lock up the lid and cook on HIGH pressure for 20 minutes

7. Release the pressure naturally and enjoy the compote!

Zucchini Cakes

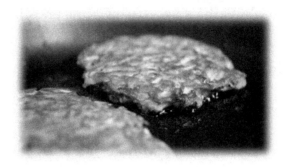

Preparation time: 10 mins

Servings: 4

Nutritional Values (Per Serving):

- Calories: 94
- Fat:1 g
- Carbs:19 g
- Protein:4 g
- Sugars:31 g
- Sodium:161 mg

Ingredients:

- Freshly ground black pepper
- 1 finely diced red onion
- 2 tsps. Salt
- 1 egg white
- Homemade horseradish sauce
- 1 shredded medium zucchini
- ¾ c. salt-free breadcrumbs

Directions:

1. Preheat oven to 400°F. Spray a baking sheet lightly with oil and set aside.
2. Press shredded zucchini gently between paper towels to remove excess liquid.
3. In a large bowl, combine zucchini, onion, egg white, breadcrumbs, seasoning, and black pepper. Mix well.
4. Shape mixture into patties and place on the prepared baking sheet.
5. Place baking sheet on middle rack in oven and bake for 10 minutes. Gently flip patties and return to oven to bake for another 10 minutes.
6. Remove from oven and serve immediately.

Two-Potato Soup with Rainbow Chard

Preparation time: 5 Minutes

Cooking time: 45 Minutes

Servings: 6

Ingredients:

- 2 tablespoons olive oil
- 1 medium red onion, chopped
- 1 medium leek, white part only, well rinsed and chopped
- 2 garlic cloves, minced
- 6 cups vegetable broth (homemade, store-bought or water)
- 1 pound red potatoes, unpeeled and cut into 1/2-inch dice
- 1 pound sweet potatoes, peeled and cut into 1/2-inch dice
- 1/4 teaspoon crushed red pepper
- Salt and freshly ground black pepper

- 1 medium bunch rainbow chard, tough stems removed and coarsely chopped

Directions:

1. In large soup pot, heat the oil over medium heat. Add the onion, leek, and garlic. Cover and cook until softened, about 5 minutes. Add the broth, potatoes, and crushed red pepper and bring to a boil. Reduce heat to low, season with salt and black pepper to taste, and simmer, uncovered, for 15 minutes.
2. Stir in the chard and cook until the vegetables are tender, about 15 minutes longer and serve.

Hot & Sour Tofu Soup

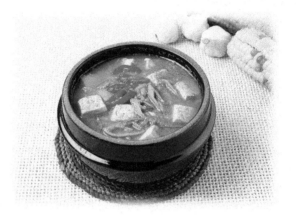

Preparation time: 40 Minutes

Cooking time: 15 Minutes

Servings: 3

Nutrition per Serving (2 cups)

- Calories: 161
- Protein: 13g
- Total fat: 9g
- Saturated fat: 1g
- Carbohydrates: 10g
- Fiber: 3g

Ingredients:

- 1 cup sliced mushrooms
- 1 cup finely chopped cabbage
- 1 garlic clove, minced
- ½-inch piece fresh ginger, peeled and minced
- Salt
- 4 cups water or Economical Vegetable Broth
- 2 tablespoons rice vinegar or apple cider vinegar
- 2 tablespoons soy sauce
- 1 teaspoon toasted sesame oil
- 1 teaspoon sugar
- Pinch red pepper flakes
- 1 scallion, white and light green parts only, chopped
- 6 to 7 ounces firm or extra-firm tofu
- 1 teaspoon olive oil

Directions:

1. Preparing the ingredients
2. Press your tofu before you start: Put it between several layers of paper towels and place a heavy pan or book (with a waterproof cover or protected with plastic wrap)

on top. Let stand for 30 minutes. Discard the paper towels. Cut the tofu into ½-inch cubes.

3. In a large soup pot, heat the olive oil over medium-high heat.

4. Add the mushrooms, cabbage, garlic, ginger, and a pinch of salt. Sauté for 7 to 8 minutes, until the vegetables are softened.

5. Add the water, vinegar, soy sauce, sesame oil, sugar, red pepper flakes, and tofu.

6. Bring to a boil, then turn the heat to low. Simmer the soup for 5 to 10 minutes.

7. Serve with the scallion sprinkled on top.

8. Leftovers will keep in an airtight container for up to 1 week in the refrigerator or up to 1 month in the freezer.

Autumn Medley Stew

Preparation time: 5 Minutes

Cooking time: 60 Minutes

Servings: 4 To 6

Ingredients:

- 2 tablespoons olive oil
- 8 ounces seitan, homemade or store-bought, cut in 1-inch cubes
- Salt and freshly ground black pepper
- 1 large yellow onion, chopped
- 2 garlic cloves, minced
- 1 large russet potato, peeled and cut into ½-inch dice
- 1 medium carrot, cut into ¼-inch dice
- 1 medium parsnip, cut into ¼-inch dice chopped
- 1 small butternut squash, peeled, halved, seeded, and cut into ½-inch dice
- 1 small head savoy cabbage, chopped
- 1 14.5-ounce can diced tomatoes, drained

- 1½ cups cooked or 1 15.5-ounce can chickpeas, drained and rinsed
- 2 cups vegetable broth,
- ½ cup dry white wine
- ½ teaspoon dried marjoram
- ½ teaspoon dried thyme
- ½ cup crumbled angel hair pasta

Directions:

1. In a large skillet, heat 1 tablespoon of the oil over medium-high heat. Add the seitan and cook until browned on all sides, about 5 minutes. Season with salt and pepper to taste and set aside.

2. In a large saucepan, heat the remaining 1 tablespoon oil over medium heat. Add the onion and garlic. Cover and cook for until softened, about 5 minutes. Add the potato, carrot, parsnip, and squash. Cover and cook until softened, about 10 minutes.

3. Stir in the cabbage, tomatoes, chickpeas, broth, wine, marjoram, thyme, and salt and pepper to taste. Bring to a boil, then reduce heat to low. Cover and cook, stirring occasionally, until the vegetables are tender, about 45 minutes.

4. Add the cooked seitan and the pasta and simmer until the pasta is tender and the flavors are blended, about 10 minutes longer. Serve immediately.
5. Variation: Leave out the pasta and serve with some warm crusty bread.

Garlic-Butter Tempeh with Shirataki Fettucine

Preparation time: 30 minutes

Serving: 4

Nutritional Values (Per Serving):

- Calories:399
- Total Fat: 34.2g
- Saturated Fat: 18.6g
- Total Carbs: 10 g
- Dietary Fiber:0g
- Sugar: 2g
- Protein:17 g
- Sodium: 283mg

Ingredients:

For the shirataki fettuccine:

- 2 (8 oz) packs shirataki fettuccine

For the garlic-butter steak bites:

- 4 tbsp butter
- 1 lb thick-cut tempeh, cut into 1-inch cubes
- Salt and black pepper to taste
- 4 garlic cloves, mined
- 2 tbsp chopped fresh parsley
- 1 cup freshly grated parmesan cheese

Directions:

For the shirataki fettuccine:

- Boil 2 cups of water in a medium pot over medium heat.
- Strain the shirataki pasta through a colander and rinse very well under hot running water.
- Allow proper draining and pour the shirataki pasta into the boiling water. Cook for 3 minutes and strain again.
- Place a dry skillet over medium heat and stir-fry the shirataki pasta until visibly dry, and makes a squeaky

sound when stirred, 1 to 2 minutes. Take off the heat and set aside.

For the garlic-butter mushroom bites:

- Melt the butter in a large skillet, season the mushroom with salt, black pepper and cook in the butter until brown, and cooked through, 10 minutes.
- Stir in the garlic and cook until fragrant, 1 minute.
- Mix in the parsley and shirataki pasta; toss well and season with salt and black pepper.
- Dish the food, top with the parmesan cheese and serve immediately.

Eggplant Ragu

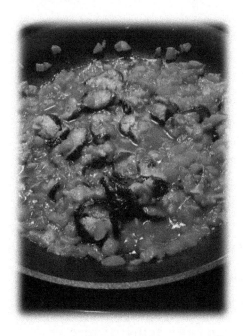

Preparation time: 20 minutes

Serving: 4

Nutritional Values (Per Serving):

- Calories: 163
- Total Fat: 9.8g
- Saturate

- Fat:5.6 g
- Total Carbs: 7 g
- Dietary Fiber:2g
- Sugar:4g
- Protein: 13g
- Sodium: 417mg

Ingredients:

- 2 tbsp butter
- 1 lb eggplant
- Salt and black pepper to taste
- 1 / 4 cup sugar-free tomato sauce
- 4 tbsp chopped fresh parsley + extra for garnishing
- 4 large green bell peppers, Blade A, noodles trimmed
- 4 large red bell peppers, Blade A, noodles trimmed
- 1 small red onion, Blade A, noodles trimmed 1 cup grated parmesan cheese

Directions:

1. Heat half of the butter in a medium skillet and cook the eggplant until brown, 5 minutes. Season with salt and black pepper.
2. Stir in the tomato sauce, parsley, and cook for 10 minutes or until the sauce reduces by a quarter.
3. Stir in the bell pepper and onion noodles; cook for 1 minute and turn the heat off.
4. Adjust the taste with salt, black pepper, and dish the food onto serving plates.
5. Garnish with the parmesan cheese and more parsley; serve warm.

Corn and Red Bean Salad

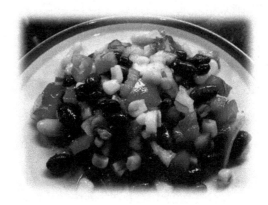

Preparation time: 10 Minutes

Cooking time: 0 Minutes

Servings: 4

Ingredients:

- 1 (10-ounce) package frozen corn kernels, cooked
- 1½ cups cooked or 1 (15.5-ounce) can dark red kidney beans, drained and rinsed
- 1 celery rib, cut into ¼-inch slices

- 2 green onions, minced
- 2 tablespoons chopped fresh cilantro or parsley
- 1/4 cup olive oil
- 2 tablespoons white wine vinegar
- 1/2 teaspoon ground cumin
- 1/4 teaspoon sugar (optional)
- 1/2 teaspoon salt (optional)
- 1/8 teaspoon freshly ground black pepper

Directions:

1. In a large bowl, combine the corn, beans, celery, green onions, and cilantro, and set aside.
2. In a small bowl, combine the oil, vinegar, cumin, sugar, salt, and pepper. Mix well and pour the dressing over the vegetables. Toss gently to combine and serve.

Greek Potato Salad

Preparation time: 10 Minutes

Cooking time: 20 Minutes

Servings: 4

Nutrition per Serving:

- Calories: 358
- Protein: 5g
- Total fat: 16g
- Saturated fat: 2g
- Carbohydrates: 52g
- Fiber: 5g

Ingredients:

- 6 potatoes, scrubbed or peeled and chopped
- Salt
- ¼ cup olive oil
- 2 tablespoons apple cider vinegar

- 2 tablespoons freshly squeezed lemon juice
- 1 teaspoon dried herbs
- ½ cucumber, chopped
- ¼ red onion, diced
- ¼ cup chopped pitted black olives
- Freshly ground black pepper

Directions:

1. Put the potatoes in a large pot, add a pinch of salt, and pour in enough water to cover. Bring the water to a boil over high heat. Cook the potatoes for 15 to 20 minutes, until soft. Drain and set aside to cool. (Alternatively, put the potatoes in a large microwave-safe dish with a bit of water. Cover and heat on high power for 10 minutes.)

2. In a large bowl, whisk together the olive oil, vinegar, lemon juice, and dried herbs. Toss the cucumber, red onion, and olives with the dressing. Add the cooked, cooled potatoes, and toss to combine. Taste and season with salt and pepper as needed. Store leftovers in an airtight container in the refrigerator for up to 1 week.

Rainbow Quinoa Salad

Preparation time: 51 Minutes

Cooking time: 0 Minutes

Servings: 6-8

Ingredients:

- 3 tablespoons olive oil
- Juice of 1½ lemons
- 1 teaspoon garlic powder
- ½ teaspoon dried oregano
- 1 bunch curly kale, stemmed and roughly chopped
- 2 cups cooked tricolor quinoa
- 1 cup canned mandarin oranges in juice, drained
- 1 cup diced yellow summer squash
- 1 red bell pepper, seeded and diced
- ½ red onion, thinly sliced
- ½ cup dried cranberries or cherries
- ½ cup slivered almonds

Directions:

1. In a small bowl, whisk together the oil, lemon juice, garlic powder, and oregano.
2. In a large bowl, toss the kale with the oil-lemon mixture until well coated. Add the quinoa, oranges, squash, bell pepper, and red onion and toss until all the **Ingredients:** are well combined. Divide among bowls or transfer to a large serving platter. Top with the cranberries and almonds.

Veggie Spread

Preparation time: 10 minutes

Cooking time: 20 minutes

Servings: 4

Nutritional Values (Per Serving):

- Calories 163
- Fat 4
- Fiber 3
- Carbs 7
- Protein 8

Ingredients:

- 2 tablespoons olive oil
- 1 cup shallots, chopped
- 2 garlic cloves, minced

- ½ cup eggplant, chopped
- ½ cup red bell pepper, chopped
- ¼ cup tomatoes, cubed
- 2 tablespoons coconut cream
- ¼ cup veggie stock
- Salt and black pepper to the taste

Directions:

1. Heat up a pan with the oil over medium heat, add the shallots and the garlic and sauté for 5 minutes.
2. Add the eggplant, tomatoes and the other ingredients, stir and cook for 15 minutes more.
3. Blend the mix a bit with an immersion blender, divide into bowls and serve cold as a party spread.

Pomegranate Dip

Preparation time: 10 minutes

Cooking time: 0 minutes

Servings: 6

Nutritional Values (Per Serving):

- Calories 294
- Fat 18
- Fiber 1
- Carbs 21
- Protein 10

Ingredients:

- 2 cups coconut cream
- 2 tablespoons walnuts, chopped
- ½ cup pomegranate seeds
- A pinch of salt and white pepper
- 2 tablespoons mint, chopped

- 2 tablespoons olive oil

Directions:

1. In a blender, combine the cream with the pomegranate seeds and the other ingredients, pulse well, divide into bowls and serve cold.

Tomato and Watermelon Bites

Preparation time: 10 minutes

Cooking time: 0 minutes

Servings: 6

Nutritional Values (Per Serving):

- Calories 162
- Fat 4
- Fiber 7
- Carbs 29
- Protein 4

Ingredients:

- 1/3 cup basil, chopped
- 1 pound cherry tomatoes, halved
- 2 cups watermelon, peeled and roughly cubed
- 1 teaspoon avocado oil
- 1 tablespoon balsamic vinegar

Directions:

In a bowl, combine the cherry tomatoes with the watermelon cubes and the other ingredients, toss, arrange on a platter and serve as an appetizer.

Artichoke and Spinach Salad

Preparation time: 5 minutes

Cooking time: 0 minutes

Servings: 4

Nutritional Values (Per Serving):

- Calories 223
- Fat 11.2
- Fiber 5.34
- Carbs 15.5
- Protein 7.4

Ingredients:

- 2 tablespoons avocado oil
- 2 garlic cloves, minced
- 2 tablespoons cilantro, chopped
- 14 ounces canned artichokes, drained and halved
- 2 cups baby spinach, chopped

- ½ cup cucumber, roughly cubed
- ½ teaspoon basil, dried
- Salt and black pepper to the taste

Directions:

In a bowl, combine the artichokes with the garlic, the oil and the other ingredients, toss, divide into smaller bowls and serve as an appetizer.

Red Pepper and Cheese Dip

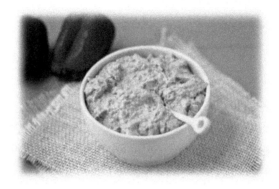

Preparation time: 10 minutes

Cooking time: 10 minutes

Servings: 4

Nutritional Values (Per Serving):

- Calories 95
- Fat 8.6
- Fiber 1.2
- Carbs 4.7
- Protein 1.4

Ingredients:

- 7 ounces roasted red peppers, chopped
- ½ cup cashew cheese, grated
- 2 tablespoons parsley, chopped
- 2 tablespoons olive oil
- ¼ cup capers, drained
- 1 tablespoon lemon juice

Directions:

2. Heat up a pan with the oil over medium heat, add the peppers and the other ingredients, stir, cook for 10 minutes and take off the heat.
3. Blend using an immersion blender, divide the mix into bowls and serve.

Mushroom Falafel

Preparation time: 10 minutes

Cooking time: 12 minutes

Servings: 6

Nutritional Values (Per Serving):

- Calories 55
- Fat 3.5
- Fiber 1.5
- Carbs 4.5
- Protein 2.3

Ingredients:

- 1 cup mushrooms, chopped
- 1 bunch parsley leaves
- 4 scallions, hopped
- 5 garlic cloves, minced
- 1 teaspoon coriander, ground

- A pinch of salt and black pepper
- ¼ teaspoon baking soda
- 1 teaspoon lemon juice
- 3 tablespoons almond flour
- 2 tablespoons avocado oil

Directions:

1. In your food processor, combine the mushrooms with the parsley and the other ingredients except the flour and the oil and pulse well.
2. Transfer the mix to a bowl, add the flour, stir well, shape medium balls out of this mix and flatten them a bit.
3. Heat up a pan with the over medium-high heat, add the falafels, cook them for 6 minutes on each side, drain excess grease using paper towels, arrange them on a platter and serve as an appetizer.

DESSERTS

Mango Rice Pudding

Preparation time: 35 Minutes

Servings: 6

Ingredients:

- 2 (14-ouncecans unsweetened coconut milk
- 2 cups unsweetened almond milk, plus more if needed
- 1 cup uncooked jasmine rice
- ½ cup granulated natural sugar, or more to taste
- 1 large ripe mango, peeled, pitted, and chopped
- 1 teaspoon coconut extract
- 1 teaspoon pure vanilla extract
- ¼ teaspoon salt

Directions:

1. Spray the Instant Pot insert with cooking spray.

2. Add the milks and bring to a boil.
3. Add the rice, sugar, and salt, seal, and cook on Rice.
4. Depressurize quickly and stir in the extracts and mango.
5. The pudding will thicken as it cools.

Tapioca with Apricots

Preparation time: 25 Minutes

Servings: 4

Ingredients:

- 2½ cups unsweetened almond milk
- ½ cup chopped dried apricots
- ⅓ cup small pearl tapioca
- ⅓ cup granulated natural sugar
- ¼ cup apricot preserves
- 1 teaspoon pure vanilla extract

Directions:

1. Spray the inside of your Instant Pot with cooking spray.
2. Put in the tapioca, sugar, almond milk, and apricots.
3. Seal and cook on Stew for 12 minutes.
4. Release the pressure fast.
5. In a bowl combine the preserve and vanilla.

6. Add the mixture to your tapioca and reseal your Instant Pot.

7. Leave to finish in its own heat.

8. Serve hot or cold.

Poached Pears in Ginger Sauce

Preparation time: 25 Minutes

Servings: 6

Ingredients:

- 2½ cups white grape juice
- 6 firm ripe cooking pears, peeled, halved, and cored
- ¼ cup natural sugar, plus more if needed
- 6 strips lemon zest
- ½ cinnamon stick
- 2 teaspoons grated fresh ginger
- Juice of 1 lemon
- Pinch of salt

Directions:

1. Warm the grape juice, ginger, lemon zest, salt, and sugar until blended.
2. Add the cinnamon stick and the pears.
3. Seal and cook on Stew for 12 minutes.

4. Take the pears out.

5. Add lemon juice and more sugar to the liquid.

6. Cook with the lid off a few minutes to thicken.

7. Serve.

Baked Apples

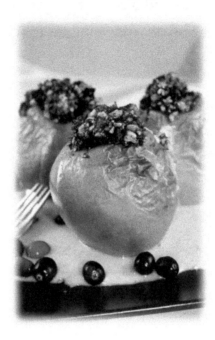

Preparation time: 35 Minutes

Servings: 6

Ingredients:

- 6 large firm Granny Smith apples, washed
- ½ cup naturally sweetened cranberry juice
- ⅓ cup sweetened dried cranberries

- ⅓ cup packed light brown sugar or granulated natural sugar
- ¼ cup crushed, chopped, or coarsely ground almonds, walnuts, or pecans
- Juice of 1 lemon
- ½ teaspoon ground cinnamon

Directions:

1. Core the apples most of the way down, leaving a little base so the stuffing stays put.
2. Stand your apples upright in your Instant Pot. Do not pile them on top of each other! You may need to do two batches.
3. In a bowl combine the sugar, nuts, cranberries, and cinnamon.
4. Stuff each apple with the mix.
5. Pour the cranberry juice around the apples.
6. Seal and cook on Stew for 20 minutes.
7. Depressurize naturally.

Maple & Rum Apples

Preparation time: 25 Minutes

Servings: 6

Ingredients:

- 6 Granny Smith apples, washed
- ½ cup pure maple syrup
- ½ cup apple juice
- ⅓ cup packed light brown sugar
- ¼ cup golden raisins
- ¼ cup dark rum or spiced rum
- ¼ cup old-fashioned rolled oats
- ¼ cup macadamia nut pieces
- 1 teaspoon ground cinnamon
- ½ teaspoon ground nutmeg
- Juice of 1 lemon

Directions:

1. Core the apples most of the way down, leaving a little base so the stuffing stays put.
2. Stand your apples upright in your Instant Pot. Do not pile them on top of each other! You may need to do two batches.
3. In a bowl combine the oats, sugar, raisins, nuts, and half the nutmeg, half the cinnamon.
4. Stuff each apple with the mix.
5. In another bowl combine the remaining nutmeg and cinnamon, the maple syrup, and the rum.
6. Pour the glaze over the apples.
7. Seal and cook on Stew for 20 minutes.
8. Depressurize naturally.

Pumpkin & Chocolate Loaf

Preparation time: 15 Minutes

Servings: 8

Ingredients:

- 1¾ cups unbleached all-purpose flour
- 1 cup canned solid-pack pumpkin
- ½ cup packed light brown sugar or granulated natural sugar
- ½ cup semisweet vegan chocolate chips
- ¼ cup pure maple syrup
- 2 tablespoons vegetable oil
- 2 teaspoons baking powder
- 1 teaspoon pure vanilla extract
- ½ teaspoon salt
- ½ teaspoon ground cinnamon
- ¼ teaspoon ground allspice
- ¼ teaspoon ground nutmeg

Directions:

1. Lightly oil a baking tray that will fit in the steamer basket of your Instant Pot.
2. In a bowl, combine the flour, baking powder, baking soda, salt and spices.
3. In another bowl combine the pumpkin, maple syrup, sugar, vanilla, and oil.
4. Stir the wet mixture into the dry mixture slowly until they form a smooth mix.
5. Fold in the chocolate chips.
6. Pour the batter into your baking tray and put the tray in your steamer basket.
7. Pour the minimum amount of water into the base of your Instant Pot and lower the steamer basket.
8. Seal and cook on Steam for 10 minutes.
9. Release the pressure quickly and set to one side to cool a little.

Cheesecake

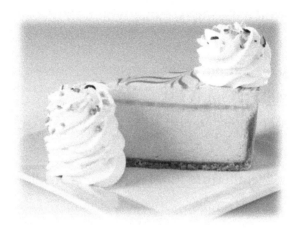

Preparation time: 45 minutes

Ingredients:

For the crust:

- 4 tbsp. butter
- 6 cups coconut, shredded
- Any sweetener you consider appropriate

For the filling:

- 8 Oz. cream cheese
- ½ cup stevia sweetener

- ½ maple syrup
- 16 Oz. can of pineapple in a syrup, crashed or whole, drained
- ¼ cup whipping cream 5 eggs

Directions:

1. After you mix all the crust ingredients press evenly and place it into the baking tray or pan and have it baked for at least 10 minutes. Let it cool.
2. In a blender mix well the cream cheese with sweeteners, the pineapple until blended.
3. Add the eggs gradually and pour this batter into the pan you have prepared.
4. Bake for 90 minutes. Remove from oven and let it cooled.

Tip: Can be served with additional pineapple on top and/or with whipped cream whatever topping you choose to your liking.

Gluten-Free Nutella Brownie Trifle

Preparation time: 60 minutes

Ingredients:

For the brownies:

- 6 Oz. hazelnuts
- ½ cup almonds
- ½ cup cashews
- 1 cup medjool dates, pitted
- ½ tsp. vanilla extract
- 2 tbsp. cacao powder
- 2 tbsp. hazelnut butter
- 1 tbsp. maple syrup or honey, to taste

For the frosting:

- ½ cup avocado, fresh crushed
- 1 ½ tbsp. coconut oil
- ½ tsp. vanilla
- 2tbsp. coconut maple syrup
- 1 tbsp. cacao

- 1 tbsp. nut butter

Directions:

1. You will need some baking paper for lining the baking tray.
2. Dry the hazelnuts and almonds in a frying pan until toasted.
3. Add ¾ of all the nuts with the almonds into the food processor until they are broken to chunks.
4. Add the dates and process again, then all the rest ingredients until you have a sticky mass.
5. Pour it onto the baking tray lined with paper. Press the crumbly mixture you made with your fingers until the top of it is even. Place into the fridge while you are cooking the glaze.
6. For the glaze you will have to mix well all the ingredients in a bowl or process them all in a food processor until well combined. It should be smooth and creamy.
7. Remove your brownie from a fridge add the frosting on top spreading it evenly.
8. Top the brownie with the remaining nuts and place again into the fridge until you have it served.

Chinese Soup and Ginger Sauce

Preparation time: 10 minutes

Cooking time: 8 hours

Servings: 6

Nutritions:

- Calories 300
- Fat 4
- Fiber 6
- Carbs 19
- Protein 4

Ingredients:

- 2 celery stalks, chopped
- 1 yellow onion, chopped
- 1 cup carrot, chopped

- 8 ounces water chestnuts
- 8 ounces canned bamboo shoots, drained
- 2 teaspoons garlic, minced
- 2 teaspoons ginger paste
- ½ teaspoon red pepper flakes
- 3 tablespoons coconut aminos
- 1-quart veggie stock
- 2 bunches bok choy, chopped
- 5 ounces white mushrooms, sliced
- 8 ounces tofu, drained and cubed
- 1 ounce snow peas, cut into small pieces
- 6 scallions, chopped

For the ginger sauce:

- 1 teaspoon sesame oil
- 2 tablespoons ginger paste
- 2 tablespoons agave syrup
- 2 tablespoon coconut aminos

Directions:

1. In your slow cooker, mix onion with carrot, celery, chestnuts, bamboo shoots, garlic paste, 2 teaspoons

ginger paste, pepper flakes, 3 tablespoons coconut aminos, stock, bok choy, mushrooms, tofu, snow peas and scallions, stir, cover and cook on Low for 8 hours.

2. In a bowl, mix 2 tablespoons ginger paste with agave syrup, 2 tablespoons coconut aminos and sesame oil and whisk well.

3. Ladle Chinese soup into bowls, add ginger sauce on top and serve.

4. Enjoy!

Corn Cream Soup

Preparation time: 10 minutes

Cooking time: 8 hours and 10 minutes

Servings: 6

Nutritions:

- Calories 312
- Fat 4
- Fiber 6
- Carbs 12
- Protein 4

Ingredients:

- 1 yellow onion, chopped
- 2 tablespoons olive oil
- 1 red bell pepper, chopped
- 3 cups gold potatoes, chopped
- 4 cups corn kernels

- 4 cups veggie stock
- ½ teaspoon smoked paprika
- 1 teaspoon cumin, ground
- Salt and black pepper to the taste
- 1 cup almond milk
- 2 scallions, chopped

Directions:

1. Heat up a pan with the oil over medium high heat, add onion, stir and cook for 5-6 minutes.
2. Transfer this to your slow cooker, add bell pepper, potatoes, 3 cups corn, stock, paprika, cumin, salt and pepper, stir, cover and cook on Low for 7 hours and 30 minutes.
3. Blend soup using an immersion blender, add almond milk and blend again.
4. Add the rest of the corn, cover pot and cook on Low for 30 minutes more.
5. Ladle soup into bowls, sprinkle scallions on top and serve.
6. Enjoy!

Veggie Medley

Preparation time: 10 minutes

Cooking time: 4 hours

Servings: 6

Nutritions:

- Calories 165
- Fat 2
- Fiber 10
- Carbs 32
- Protein 9

Ingredients:

- 1 tablespoon ginger, grated
- 3 garlic cloves, minced
- 1 date, pitted and chopped
- 1 and ½ teaspoon coriander, ground
- ½ teaspoon dry mustard

- 1 and ¼ teaspoon cumin, ground
- A pinch of salt and black pepper
- ½ teaspoon turmeric powder
- 1 tablespoon white wine vinegar
- ¼ teaspoon cardamom, ground
- 2 carrots, chopped
- 1 yellow onion, chopped
- 4 cups cauliflower florets
- 1 and ½ cups kidney beans, cooked
- 2 zucchinis, chopped
- 6 ounces tomato paste
- 1 green bell pepper, chopped
- 1 cup green peas

Directions:

1. In your slow cooker, mix ginger with garlic, date, coriander, dry mustard, cumin, salt, pepper, turmeric, vinegar, cardamom, carrots, onion, cauliflower, kidney beans, zucchinis, tomato paste, bell pepper and
2. peas, stir, cover and cook on High for 4 hours.
3. Divide into bowls and serve hot.
4. Enjoy!

Lentils Curry

Preparation time: 10 minutes

Cooking time: 6 hours

Servings: 8

Nutritions:

- Calories 105
- Fat 1
- Fiber 7
- Carbs 22
- Protein 7

Ingredients:

- 10 ounces spinach
- 2 cups red lentils
- 1 tablespoon garlic, minced
- 15 ounces canned tomatoes, chopped
- 2 cups cauliflower florets

- 1 teaspoon ginger, grated
- 1 yellow onion, chopped
- 4 cups veggie stock
- 2 tablespoons curry paste
- ½ teaspoon cumin, ground
- ½ teaspoon coriander, ground
- 2 teaspoons stevia
- A pinch of salt and black pepper
- ¼ cup cilantro, chopped
- 1 tablespoon lime juice

Directions:

1. In your slow cooker, mix spinach with lentils, garlic, tomatoes, cauliflower, ginger, onion, stock, curry paste, cumin, coriander, stevia, salt, pepper and lime juice, stir, cover and cook on Low for 6 hours.
2. Add cilantro, stir, divide into bowls and serve.
3. Enjoy!

Lentils Dal

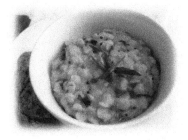

Preparation time: 10 minutes

Cooking time: 5 hours

Servings: 12

Nutritions:

- Calories 283
- Fat 4
- Fiber 8
- Carbs 12
- Protein 4

Ingredients:

- 6 cups water

- 3 cups red lentils
- 28 ounces canned tomatoes, chopped
- 1 yellow onion, chopped
- 4 garlic cloves, minced
- 1 tablespoon turmeric powder
- 2 tablespoons ginger, grated
- 3 cardamom pods
- 1 bay leaf
- 2 teaspoons mustard seeds
- 2 teaspoons onion seeds
- 2 teaspoons fenugreek seeds
- 1 teaspoon fennel seeds
- Salt and black pepper to the taste

Directions:

1. In your slow cooker, mix water with lentils, tomatoes, onion, garlic, turmeric, ginger, cardamom, bay leaf, mustard seeds, onion seeds, fenugreek seeds, fennel seeds, salt and pepper, stir, cover and cook on High for 5 hours.
2. Divide into bowls and serve.
3. Enjoy!

Fruit Dish

Preparation time: 10 minutes

Cooking time: 6 hours

Servings: 4

Nutritions:

- calories 160
- fat 4
- fiber 1
- carbs 20
- protein 4

Ingredients:

- ½ cup tamari
- 40 ounces canned young jackfruit, drained
- ¼ cup coconut aminos 1 cup mirin
- ½ cup agave nectar
- 8 garlic cloves, minced

- 2 tablespoons ginger, grated
- 1 yellow onion, chopped
- 4 tablespoons sesame oil
- 1 green pear, cored and chopped
- ½ cup water

Directions:

1. In your slow cooker, mix tamari with jackfruit, aminos, mirin, agave nectar, garlic, ginger, onion, sesame oil, water and pear, stir, cover and cook on Low for 6 hours.
2. Divide into bowls and serve.
3. Enjoy!